Pre-Diabetes Warning Signs: Proven Tips How to Reverse the Early Symptoms

Table of content

Introduction

When people think of diabetes, they sometimes imagine daily injections of insulin, a complete removal of all sugary foods from the diet and frightening physical symptoms such as blackouts, damage to vision and amputation. If you have been diagnosed as prediabetic, please do not panic. You have been notified that Type 2 diabetes is in your future unless you take steps now to halt or slow down its onset. Although diabetes can be a serious, chronic, life-limiting condition, there is a lot you can do to mitigate its effects.

Now is the time to take some decisive action to safeguard your health. It may seem daunting but there are many avenues of support out there for you which can help you achieve your goals. Later on we will discuss in more detail the myriad of options for losing weight and increasing fitness that there are out there, but for now just know that there are many possibilities for you to explore, and that you can find the one that is right for you.

Even a 5 per cent reduction in body fat is thought to drop your chances of going on to develop diabetes by 50 per cent. You may have intended for a while to make changes to your health and fitness; use your diagnosis as the perfect motivational tool. Now is the time — the time when you make the choice to improve your health and take control of your condition.

Chapter 1 – What is Prediabetes?

Prediabetes is sometimes called 'borderline diabetes' and it is a condition in which you have higher than normal blood glucose levels, but which are not yet high enough to be termed diabetes itself. A FPGT (Fasting Plasma Glucose Test) result of 6 or below is normal, between 6 and 7 indicates prediabetes and a result of 7 and above confirms diabetes*.

It is strongly linked to obesity and carries the risk of becoming Type 2 Diabetes in the future. It is estimated that up to 7 million people in the UK have prediabetes, but numbers are hard to gauge since so many people are unaware that they are at risk. Symptoms develop gradually and can only begin to show once the person has passed the prediabetic stage.

However, at the prediabetic stage it is possible to slow down the onset of Type 2 diabetes or even eliminate it entirely.

Type 2 diabetes is a condition in which the body has a high blood sugar level, either because of insulin resistance or a relative lack of insulin. Insulin is produced by the body to turn sugar in the blood into glycogen, which can then be safely stored by the body. Insulin resistance is when the muscles, liver and fatty tissue stop responding adequately to the effects of insulin and can no longer regulate the levels of sugar in the blood.

Type 2 is different from Type 1 diabetes, which is a condition where the body produces no insulin at all, due to damage of the pancreas. Type 1 cannot be controlled by lifestyle changes and requires treatment with insulin. Type 2 can also be managed with medication, but the effects can be reduced or managed with lifestyle changes.

*These figures are in millimoles per liter, often abbreviated to mmol/l

Chapter 2 – Risk Factors

There are a number of factors which may increase your risk of developing prediabetes. These are:

* Being overweight or obese
* Being aged 40 or over
* Having a close relative who has already developed diabetes
* Have given birth to a baby weighing over 9 pounds
* Having high blood pressure
* Having a sedentary life with little or no exercise

There is also evidence that people from some ethnic backgrounds are more at risk from prediabetes. These groups are :

* South Asian (Type 2 diabetes is up to six times more likely to develop)
* Native American
* Afro-Caribbean (Type 2 diabetes is up to three times more likely to develop)

Obesity is the number one cause of prediabetes and is on the increase due to changes in diet and lifestyle. As more and more people work in sedentary jobs their daily calorie requirement decreases, as well as having less time and fewer facilities for exercise. At the same time, the prevalence of high-sugar, high-fat and low-fibre foods mean that it is easy to consume more than your body requires.

It also seems to make a difference how your fat is distribute around your body. People who carry excess weight around their tummy are at higher risk than people whose fat is distributed more evenly over their body, or predominantly on the hips and thighs. A larger waist size is a more reliable way to determine your risk than measuring your BMI, since BMI can be affected by muscle mass. As a general rule, a waist measurement of more than 94cm (37 inches) for men or 80cm (32.5 inches) for women is considered at risk.

Chapter 3 – Symptoms of Prediabetes

The symptoms of prediabetes can be hard to spot, since it develops gradually and often does not present any outward signs at all until diabetes has developed. However, there may be some signs, including:

- Thirst. People who are developing diabetes often find themselves ragingly thirsty and drinking a lot more water and soft beverages than they usually would.

- Frequent urination or large volumes of very dilute urine. This is unsurprising if the person is also drinking a lot of water, but points to the thirst as not being due to dehydration.

- Fatigue.

- Increased hunger coupled with weight loss.

- Other more uncommon symptoms include blurred vision, itchy skin, increased fungal infections (such as thrush) and tingling in the hands and feet.

Many people who are diagnosed with Type 2 diabetes have not experienced significant symptoms, however and find out their diagnosis after a routine test. You are very unlikely to have suffered from a blood sugar 'low' which causes faintness, disorientation and sometimes unconsciousness and which many people think of as one of the 'classic' symptom of diabetes.

The best way to tell if you have prediabetes is with a blood test which your GP can administer. You can ask to have this done routinely, especially if you are at risk from more than one factor. There are two main types of test which are used:

Fasting Plasma Glucose Test: this test measures the levels of glucose in your blood. In order for the result to be accurate it is import to not eat or drink anything except water for eight hours beforehand. It requires a quick finger-prick to obtain a small amount of blood.

Oral Glucose Tolerance Test: this test is the same as the FPGT, except that after fasting for eight hours, you are given a drink with a specific amount of glucose in it. Your blood sugar is then measured at intervals to see how quickly your body copes with the new glucose in your system.

For both methods, the results will usually be confirmed with a follow-up test on a different day.

A doctor can also measure your blood sugar level on the spot, without you needing to fast beforehand, however this test is only useful of detecting diabetes, not prediabetes.

Chapter 4 – Reducing your risk.

If you have one or more of the risk factors associated with prediabetes, ask you GP for a test. If it comes back that you have already developed prediabetes, there are a number of things you can do to delay the onset of diabetes or even stop it altogether.

The number one thing you can do to improve your health is to reduce your body fat and increase your fitness.

Also consider reducing your alcohol intake — as well as contributing 'empty' calories, increased consumption of alcohol is linked to an increasing risk of diabetes.

Think about any causes of stress in your life. We will discuss stress in more detail in chapter 8, but it is important to think of ways to eliminate or reduce stress in your life. Going for a walk, meditation or a bath are all simple ways to help you relax.

Increase the amount of fiber in your diet. As well as making you feel fuller, fiber has been shown to absorb cholesterol in the gut. Higher cholesterol has also been linked to increased risk of diabetes as well as heart disease and strokes.

NB: If you have a low-fiber diet to begin with, introduce more fiber gradually and build up the levels over time. It can cause bloating, discomfort, wind and diarrhea to suddenly go from no fiber to a high level, so don't suddenly start taking fiber supplements or eating bran.

Although no one is entirely sure exactly why the link exists, there are several theories to explain why being overweight can cause diabetes:

- When a cell has more nutrients and energy than it can process, it shuts down the insulin receptors on its surface. Over time, this leads to the cell becoming 'resistant' in that it no longer correctly responds to the presence of insulin.

- Changes to your metabolism (such as being overweight) cause fat molecules to be released into the blood stream. The fat molecules enter muscle and liver cells and damage the cell's ability to respond to insulin.

- Carrying excess fat around the middle of your body (a so-called 'spare tyre') is especially damaging since abdominal fat cells can release 'pro-inflammatory' chemicals which are linked to insulin resistance in cells.

All of these theories agree that the more fatty tissue you have in your body, the more likely you are to suffer from diabetes, and that the best way to reduce your risk is to lose weight.

Chapter 5 – Losing Weight

There are a million and one products, regimes and philosophies out there, all promising fast, permanent weight loss. You may have already tried a few yourself, and have a good idea of the upsides and downsides of the various methods.

We cannot promise to tell you the weight loss method that is right for you, however there are a few things to bear in mind to help youmake the most of your weight loss journey.

An important thing to do is to set a main goal and then decide on a series of smaller, achievable milestones that will lead towards it. A good starting point might be to decide to lose 5 per cent of your bodyweight. Your GP can support you in your weight loss by setting reasonable goals, providing you with information and monitoring your progress. Or he or she might refer you to a specialist health program for people attempting to lose weight.

All pills, supplements, herbals teas and 'natural remedies' that you can buy over the counter or on the internet are ineffective. At best, they are simply laxatives. At worst, they can be dangerous. Please steer clear of anything promising 'instant' weight loss or miraculous progress — a pill that makes you thin with no side effects is the holy grail of the pharmaceutical industry, and it has not been found yet.

Many people find that slimming groups are beneficial. The majority of the success seems to come from the weekly weigh-ins and group support which is available to you. If you don't fancy a slimming group, you could maybe team up with a friend or partner to support each other.

Especially for the first few weeks, it is extremely helpful to keep a food diary. Make sure you honestly write down everything you eat — it can be very easy for snacks and add-ons to slip your mind. You aren't going to show this to anybody, so don't worry about what someone would think if they saw it. This is just for you. It can also help you to keep an eye on your portion sizes. It's very easy to dish out more food than you need, especially if we are comparing what should be on our plates to the volumes served in restaurants or those around us.

There are lots of websites and apps available which can allow you to track your progress as well as letting you put in your food consumption, exercise and weight. Check reviews online or ask a friend for a recommendation. Some people find these suit them very well, especially if they give visual markers of your progress. Watching a line on a graph go down and down can be very satisfying.

Although most people think of weight loss as something you measure with a scale, it is just as good to keep track of how many inches you are losing from your body. Especially with prediabetes, you could take your waist measurement and decide to have as your goal reducing it to under the size indicated as a risk factor. Measurements can be more reliable than pounds as they are less affected by things like dehydration, time of day and daily fluctuations — weighing yourself every day does not always give an accurate picture. If you do choose to weigh yourself, you should aim for one 'official' weigh-in at the same time each week. (Although of course you can weigh yourself in between those times if you need more motivation.)

The average amount of weight loss to aim for is 2 pounds per week. This is a safe, sustainable level of weight loss and reduces the risks of 'yo-yo' dieting. You may find that you lose weight more easily in the beginning, which can give you a boost of confidence and spur you on to keep going. Later, you may find your weight loss slowing or even halting for a week or so. If this happens, review your food diary to make sure that extra calories haven't crept in, increase your exercise levels and hang in there. You have done so well on your weight-loss journey; this is just a bump in the road.

Very restrictive diets, meal replacement foods (like shakes or soups) and intermittent fasting patterns can be effective in the short term, although it is important not to simply revert to your usual eating habits once they are over. Otherwise you will just find yourself putting the weight back on, and you will have to put yourself through the whole process again. However, they can be useful for kick-starting weight loss and providing a boost to motivation. Just make sure you have a plan for how you are going to sustain your weight loss when you come off them. Being on a very restrictive diet long-term can lead to nutrient deficiencies, food intolerances and other health problems, so only use them for short periods and make sure that you also adjust your 'normal' diet to include a balanced range of foods. Fats, carbohydrates and proteins are all good foods — it's just the proportion in your diet and the sources you choose that matter.

NB: Steer clear of 'juice fasts' or diets where you only drink water for long periods. These are very severe, can make it hard to function day-to-day and you are very likely to regain the weight once you start eating again.

Chapter 6 — Increasing your fitness

One of the best ways to support your weight loss is through regular exercise. Not only do you burn calories while you exercise, but your metabolism continues to operate at a higher level for at least 4 hours after you stop. You will develop lean muscle, which has a greater calorie requirement than fat and so means that your body will burn more energy even when you are resting. Exercise helps with regulation of mood and can also be enjoyable.

Some people (who have found it hard to stick to an exercise regime in the past) think that if they join an expensive gym they will then 'have' to go so as not to waste the money. In reality, this leads to guilt and wasted cash. If you have not in the past been a regular gym goer, some good advice before you sign up is to set yourself a program of exercises to do in your own home for three weeks. These can be simple — sit-ups and press-ups are some of the best moves to increase your strength and work major muscles groups. Make yourself a program of exercises (there are any number of fitness videos available free of charge on the internet) and decide to do them at least three times a week. Factor in a run or brisk walk at least once a week. If after three weeks you have been able to stick to your program, you can consider joining a gym. If you find that you are making excuses to miss sessions, shorten them or that you have lost enthusiasm, then the likelihood is that you would not make best use of your gym membership and need to find another avenue for physical exercise.

One of the best ways to increase your activity levels is to walk more. This will save you money (on petrol, bus fares and so on) as well as saving you time — a forty minute walk instead of a fifteen minute car journey means that you have got forty minutes of exercise at a cost of only twenty five extra minutes of your time. If you commute to work in rush hour, it can actually be quicker (or about the same) to walk to work. If you are used to commuting for an hour through a city, think about how much ground you could cover in that time, as well as maybe being able to take a more direct route. This also means that exercise will become part of your lifestyle, rather than an 'extra' that exists outside of your routine.

Running is another great, cheap way to increase your fitness. All you need are a pair of trainers and a decent sports bra (if you require one). It is not necessary to spend a large amount of money on specialist running shoes; in the beginning you are unlikely to be covering long distances and will not require them. (If you enjoy running and find yourself running further and further, you can invest in new shoes.) There are online tools which allow you to map out routes around your house of varying lengths as well as free podcasts and apps which give you set periods of time to run for, gradually increasing the distances until you are running continuously for half an hour.

If you prefer to exercise with other people there are lots of options to consider. You could start taking dancing classes (many places offer 'complete beginner' sessions) or do a fitness session which includes dance moves. You could learn to box (this is great for men and women), try a racket sport or start swimming. If you have a local sports centre or library, look on the notice board to see if there are amateur teams in your area looking for new members — football, netball, hockey and so on. If you aren't sure what you might enjoy, try a number of different types of exercise and see what suits you best. Is there something you have always wanted to try?

NB There is no need to invest a lot of money in expensive equipment. If you are doing something that requires specific kit, go to a place that will allow you to borrow the equipment you need until you are sure the sport is for you. You can then start gradually amassing your own kit.

Chapter 7 — Setting Goals

As with all endeavors, you should set yourself achievable goals. Make you first goal something that you can reasonably achieve in six to eight weeks; say a loss of twelve pounds or being able to run a mile. Check with your doctor before embarking on a lifestyle overhaul and discuss with him or her what it is that you intend to do. Your doctor may offer advice or book a follow up visit to check things like cholesterol and blood pressure which it can be difficult to monitor at home.

Then break your goal down into weekly milestones. It might look like this:

Week 1: Take your starting weight and make yourself a wall chart of your progress. You can do this in the form of a graph, or just a list of figures. Find three slots in the week of an hour which you can dedicate to fitness. Write them in your diary or set an alarm on your phone. Start keeping a food diary.

Week 2: Review your food diary and see if you can spot where your particular triggers are. If you ate more than you wanted to or did not eat healthily, see if there is a pattern; were you bored, in a rush or upset? Think of strategies that could help you cope in the future — if you eat unhealthily because you don't have time to cook, can you prepare and freeze some healthy meals in advance? Weight yourself again (or take your measurements) and add them to the chart.

Week 3: Review your exercise regime. You find that you are increasing in strength and fitness, but if you find you are becoming demotivated, try to think about why that might be. Perhaps you need to push yourself a bit harder to get the results you want. Weight yourself again (or take your measurements) and add them to the chart.

Week 4: The halfway stage. You should have lost around 6 pounds and be able to participate more fully in your chosen sport. If this hasn't happened, think about why that might be. Perhaps you need to increase your exercise sessions or eat more healthily.

Week 5: This is a good time to give an extra push. By the end of week 6 you should have achieved your goal, so tell yourself you're going to go all out this week to succeed. Think of a reward for yourself when you have reached your goal — that could be a night out with friends, a new article of clothing, a trip to the cinema, whatever would motivate you.

NB: Try not to use food as a motivation. If you think 'when I've lost six pounds I can have a sausage roll' then you may be linking food and reward in your head. If you want a sausage roll, think of a menu for the day that would mean all the fat and calories could be offset by the other foods you ate (so the rest of your day comprised only low calorie foods) so that you do not overeat on that day. You are allowed the sausage roll — you just have to budget for it.

Week 6: At the end of week six, review your progress. If you have achieved your goal, celebrate! You have done very well and should feel proud of yourself. Write your final weight on your chart and set yourself a new goal for the next six weeks.

If you haven't achieved your goal, don't let it discourage you. Review your food diary and exercise plan, and see if you can spot what might have gone wrong. See if there were 'danger spots' where you found it harder to stick to your plan and think of ways to improve them. Give yourself a further two weeks to reach your target, and then set a new goal.

Chapter 8 — Stress

Stress, both physical and emotional, has an important part to play in managing your prediabetes. Stress can encourage the production of cortisol which changes your blood sugar levels. Stress can also make it harder to adjust to a new diet and exercise regime.

It may be very worrying and upsetting to find out you have prediabetes. You may feel anxious about the future, or embarrassed that your lifestyle has caused your health to suffer. You may worry about what it means for your family or whether you will be able to manage a lifelong chronic condition.

You may also be experiencing external stress in your day-to-day life. The pace of modern life can be very hectic and many people will experience financial, marital, family or work-related stress in their lifetime.

To cope with any stress caused by your diagnosis, there are a wide range of sources that can help you work out the best way to manage your condition. The more you find out and understand what is happening to your body, the more in control you will feel and the easier it will be to reduce or resolve your symptoms. There are also support groups, both online and face-to-face, where you can meet other people who have been through the same thing and can offer advice and support.

Exercise is a great stress-buster, and has been found to be as effective as mild medication to help with low mood. Along with the physical benefits you will experience, many people find exercise also has psychological benefits.

If you feel you are suffering from stress, you should take that feeling seriously. Ask for help for friends or family, and see if there are practical steps you can take to alleviate any external factors which are worrying you. If you feel constantly on edge, tearful or despairing, you should mention this to your GP. He or she will not judge you, and will have seen many people before who are also suffering in this way. Your doctor will be able to suggest some things which will help — don't feel worried that he or she will simply 'put you on antidepressants'. These are only one of a range of treatments your doctor might suggest, and it would be completely up to you if you wanted to take them. You deserve to feel well and happy, and you don't have to do it all on your own.

Many people with Type 2 diabetes are able to turn their lives around and manage or entirely eliminate their symptoms. With dedication, information and support, you will be one of those people.

Chapter 9 – Treatments for Diabetes

If you do go on to develop diabetes, there are a number of treatments which can manage your condition, although as yet there is no cure.

The number one treatment for Type 2 diabetes is still by making lifestyle changes to lose weight and increase fitness levels. There are some medications that your doctor can prescribed to manage your condition. They work in a number of different ways:

- To stop the liver from producing more glucose

- To aid in overcoming insulin resistance.

- To stimulate the pancreas to produce more insulin

- To help the insulin that is produced to work more effectively

- To slow down the absorption of starchy foods from the intestine and so prevent spikes in blood sugar

You may be prescribed a combination of drugs, some of which are swallowed in tablets or in solution, or sometimes administered via injection. However, for Type 2 diabetes it is very unlikely that you will require daily shots of insulin, which many people think of as the 'typical' treatment for diabetes.

If left untreated or not properly managed, diabetes can shorten your life expectancy by ten years. You are more likely to suffer from heart problems, stroke and kidney problems. There is also a much higher risk of blindness (caused by high blood sugar damaging the flow of blood to the retina of the eye) and amputation of lower limbs (due to lack of blood flow).

If you have diabetes, it is extremely important to have yearly foot checks carried out by a doctor or nurse. Diabetes can gradually damage the nerves, meaning that you may not even feel pain from a developing ulcer. You should also get into the habit of checking your own feet every day. If you notice any damage — such as bruising, missing skin, blisters, sores or ulcers, get them checked out by a doctor as soon as possible. By doing so you are giving yourself the best possible chance of healing quickly and fully.

Conclusion

We hope you have enjoyed this book. Although Type 2 diabetes is a serious condition, there is no need for it to be a frightening one. If you have been diagnosed as prediabetic then this will be the warning sign you need to motivate you. You can improve your health and fitness, watch what you eat, have regular check ups and live a normal, healthy, happy life. Some people, by taking prompt and committed action, are able to reverse the effects of prediabetes so that they never develop the full condition.

There are many sources of information out there — support groups, online literature, organizations, your GP or health worker — which can help you continue to learn about your condition and improve your health.